Table of Contents

Dispelling Birth Control Myths: Uncovering the Facts and Essential Information

1. Introduction to Birth Control Myths

Birth control methods refer to contraceptives or devices used to slow down, prevent, or reduce the chances of pregnancy. According to the WHO, family planning allows individuals and couples to anticipate and attain their goals in terms of the number of children they have and the spacing and time in which they want those children. The use of birth control is not limited to the typical family, however, it is worn or ingested by couples for various purposes. Now that we have a general understanding of birth control and the negative influences of common myths, it is time to pull back the curtain. The following are the most common myths or a list of notes everyone should know to be more aware of birth control in an overall manner.

Birth control methods and family planning remain a stigmatized topic throughout the world. Despite social progress, it is common for individuals to shudder at the thought of "birth control" as if talking about it may bring the idea into existence. To compound the situation, rumors and myths surround the birth control topic. These myths hold so much power that anyone speaking of them is often met with skepticism or even outright anger. However, the best way to attack these stigmas is by sharing the facts. By doing so, individuals can be empowered to make informed decisions regarding their body, and according to the World Health Organization (WHO), empowered individuals are more likely to contribute to the growth and development in their communities and country.

1.1. Understanding the Importance of Accurate Information

On January 24th, 2021, I instrumentalized a training of 35 people, including women and men, to challenge this myth so that service providers are equipped to give full information on contraception and debunk a myth. First, people need to understand how a method works to make a correct choice and avoid misconceptions like "it's better to not use anything because they all make one infertile" or "I don't need to use contraception because I will die anyway if it is me to live." Thinking of family planning, some bring up the issue of compromised cervix. Men need to understand what this means and dispel the myth because it is holding them back from seeking an alternative method. The more we can provide correct information on contraceptive methods, the more we will create demand for family planning. We need to address misconceptions around birth control methods and give a balanced view to enable informed choice. Making it clear that it's not a health worker or someone else's choice. It's their choice to live how they want, and it's our job to give information so that they can make a choice if they want to quit pregnancy or not.

When considering birth control methods, it is indeed important to have accurate information since any misinformation or myths may carry a significant impact on personal choice. There are many misconceptions about birth control methods. Pregnant on the pill, can't get pregnant if sex is in water or standing up, birth control =

abortion, use of birth control is against some religion, types of birth control that lead to infertility, condoms are not effective in preventing pregnancy, withdrawal method is effective in preventing pregnancy, breastfeeding can prevent pregnancy, LARCs can cause weight gain, LARCs can cause infertility are some examples. Most of the misconceptions about birth control methods are rooted in more than just information. The underlying issue is social beliefs and stigmatizations deeply rooted in society. You could walk into a clinic and get information, but what you do not hear are the societal conversations about various types of birth control. Therefore, it is important to dispel the information when the need arises.

2. Historical Context of Birth Control

In the 19th and 20th centuries, orthodox criticism against contraception began to soften, and birth control techniques from different countries (primarily Asia or Africa) made their way into the western world. The development of diaphragms by 1880 inspired five different sperm-killing jelly experiments: the combination actually made good sense; women disliked spermicidal jellies, and so the diaphragm was combined with a shot, an amount of sea sponge, and finally a piece of condom-like rubber manufactured by Julius Schmid. With the birth of rubber cap diaphragms and IUDs came studies and attempts at hormonal methods. Most of these failed, including early forms of the pill, until the discovery of early IUD pains and the modification of principles. By 1960, female-controlled hormonal methods were announced.

Birth control options known to early societies often took on a dubious image. Women attempting to protect themselves from pregnancy frequently ingested poisonous or toxic substances under the belief that these items warded off pregnancies or instigated spontaneous abortion. The herbs of Silphium and Pennyroyal, used as early as 300 B.C., are both believed to have been utilized for this purpose. The more formal aspect of birth control came when mercury was identified as a cause of sterility and the first efforts to create male contraceptives were made. When using condoms (made of animal intestines) and sponges were rejected by traditional societies, male and female barrier methods failed to gain popularity for roughly 2,000 years.

2.1. Evolution of Birth Control Methods

In ancient and medieval world societies, children carried and delivered the mother's inheritance, represented a supporting workforce, or fulfilled productive gender roles themselves (in addition to those of possible mothers and wives), and multiplication has remained an economic priority. In the 18th and 19th-century industrial classes of mainland Europe and the United States, however, industrialization introduced urbanization and aroused classism and corvee attitudes toward children. Some postpartum women desired an effective means to prevent pregnancy shortly after the infancy. Evolutionarily, "neoteny" - or the juvenilization of a lineage by slow classical natural selection - also increases the relative proportion of organisms who survive gory childbirths, but other women have not desired to be prevented from "suddenly" evolving adult characters like quite possibly ages of the evolutionary selective epidemics of puberty and regular ovulation. From these circumstances, a woman who discovered the postpartum anovulation that increases keratinized human afterbirths can prevent the further exhausting burden of another pregnancy resulting in attending at least one premenstrual period, a vaginal diet, and a "hormonal sleeplessness" drink, each of which we explore after placing them in a historic context. Upstate New York postparturient women launched the first widespread American puerperal "missing solution" in their nationally-imitated Restore-The-Senses movement.

Rhythm, calendar method, and withdrawal. When convincing a partner about the necessity of prevention, few women had legal alternatives.

Dispelling birth control myths: Uncovering the facts and essential information that you need.

3. Types of Birth Control Methods

1. Hormonal methods - These birth control methods primarily involve delivering estrogen and progestin hormones. They are used to override and regulate the menstrual cycle to help women avoid pregnancy based upon irregular timing of ovulation. 2. Barrier methods - Condoms, the female condom (internal condom), diaphragms, cervical caps, and some types of sponges are all barrier methods that are used in the male and/or female to prevent semen from entering the uterus. 3. LARCs (long-acting reversible contraceptives) - LARCs are very effective at preventing pregnancy; they are placed inside a woman's uterus after counseling with her healthcare provider. 4. Natural methods - These methods allow a woman to track her fertility, mostly consisting of the days in the menstrual cycle when unprotected intercourse should be avoided to prevent pregnancy.

If you are interested in birth control as a method of contraception to prevent pregnancy, then there are a variety of methods available that can assist you. Birth control methods are often divided into four categories, depending on how they work and how they are used. The four categories are hormonal methods, barrier methods, LARCs (long-acting reversible contraceptives), and natural methods. You may be able to choose from a variety of birth control methods, including different methods from within a category and different categories of birth control. The method selected may be influenced by a combination of personal preferences as well as health considerations. Doctors can often discuss your options and provide advice to help you determine which method may be best for you.

3.1. Hormonal Methods

Hormonal contraceptives work by stopping the release of an egg – ovulation. They also thicken the mucus around the cervix, which can stop sperm getting through. They don't protect against STIs. Also known as "the pill", oral contraceptives contain man-made hormones. When taken in directed doses, these hormones prevent an egg from being released and also thicken the mucus around the cervix, making it hard for sperm to get through. As a result, ovulation is effectively stopped and sperm is hindered from reaching the uterus and fallopian tubes. Hormonal contraceptives are currently the most reliable birth control pills. These can either contain both estrogen and progestin, or just progestin. Any birth control pill containing just progestin, and not estrogen, is also called the minipill. Hormonal methods are especially popular in many countries and experts believe in theory, and important contraceptive pill can prevent pregnancies. It should, in any case, improve contraceptive methods.

The term "hormonal methods" usually refers to the category of birth control methods that contain hormones as the main ingredient. Combined hormonal contraceptive methods used daily: the pill, the patch, and the ring. With the blacklist of most pills in some countries, should one then regularly use contraception with hormones? Use of hormonal contraception – no proof. Contraception according to the contraceptive pill only requires sexual intercourse during the week of tablets with placebo. But contraception according to the pill can only be counted as effective in preventing pregnancy if couples have sex only during this period. Therefore, you are not protected from pregnancy. There are, of course, other risks.

Myth: I do not need to use a contraceptive because withdrawal is effective. Fact: Withdrawal is also known as "coitus interruptus," and it can be performed by the man or woman to avoid a potentially pregnancy-causing stigma. Pulling out is simply removing a flaccid penis from a vaginal canal before ejaculation—or ceasing oral sex before parturition. This is not a conducive approach. Even though withdrawal can protect against insemination, it is less effective than the consistent and correct use of other contraceptive methods. In fact, withdrawal is often not used powerfully or at all. Without withdrawal, sperm have the potential to infiltrate the vaginal mucus, thereby causing insemination. This brings the method's effectiveness down to approximately a 1 in 5 chance, or 22% failure rate.

For some individuals, a barrier method of birth control may be a good prescription, both to alleviate physical discomfort associated with other birth control methods and also to inhibit the spread of sexually transmitted infections. Barrier methods include condoms for both males and females as well as contraceptive sponges. These methods physically (i.e., through the use of a barrier) and chemically block sperm from reaching and fertilizing an egg. Barrier methods are one of the least effective forms of contraception with a 71-73% effectiveness. This is mostly due to both incorrect use (e.g. not using a condom the whole time, not using it from the start to finish of intercourse) and failure (e.g. a condom breaking).

3.3. Long-Acting Reversible Contraceptives (LARCs)

One of the biggest misconceptions we hear about LARCs is that they are only for people that have given birth. Not true. Teens, people in their twenties, and individuals who have never given birth can safely use LARCs. Physically, we actually know less about the big impact of pregnancy on adolescents and young adults than we do in older adults, but what we do know is that pregnancies in teenagers are more likely to be complicated by anemia, pre-eclampsia/eclampsia, and pre-term delivery. As with most contraception, the best fitting method varies from person to person and therefore a healthcare provider should discuss the potential methods available to you, along with options that you think would best fit your lifestyle, and help make a decision from there. With the exception of sterilization, the majority of other birth control methods are reversible. Most people find that there is weird timing with bleeding patterns for the first 3 to 12 months after a LARC is first inserted. Over this time, most people have less bleeding and about 1 in 3 people stop getting their period. After the adjustment period, a small number of people will begin to experience more spotting. Many people with LARC say that these bleeding changes are one of the best parts of using these methods because they interfere less with everyday life and are typically much lighter than their natural bleeding pattern. Modern IUDs also contain a small amount of hormone that primarily works in the uterus, but also prevents the egg from being released from the ovary each month. The hormone in an IUD can also thicken cervical mucus, making it harder for sperm to swim into the uterus. The hormone in an IUD continues working very effectively at this spot as well for many years. If you and a healthcare provider determine the right LARC for you, they will insert it into your uterus or arm. Most people find the insertion process fairly quick, and about a minute of cramping or pressure immediately afterwards. Because of the risk of STIs and PID, some healthcare providers might recommend having a LARC inserted after testing for and treating STIs. Want to know the best part? When you're ready to get pregnant, you'll be able to do so as quickly as if you hadn't used a LARC at all.

Long-acting reversible contraceptives (LARCs) are IUDs and implants that you wouldn't need to think about for at least 3 years and up to 12 years, depending on the LARC. Once inserted, they offer amazing protection from pregnancy. Less than 1 in 100 people will get pregnant over a year of using a LARC. This might sound a bit like a magic trick, but it's not—it's just birth control. Once removed, LARCs don't affect your long-term fertility. Long-acting reversible contraceptives are for anyone who might want long-term pregnancy protection and is comfortable with not having to think about pregnancy prevention every day.

3.4. Natural Methods

Myths: Natural methods are not safe enough for secure protection from pregnancy. Spending the necessary time required for Fertility Awareness Methods each day is not realistic. Women cannot protect themselves from pregnancies in certain situations with natural contraceptive methods. A couple faced with the decision to stop using birth control methods surely is: they do not wish to have children yet (at all) but it is the wrong time for a child. The understanding of safe/birth control automatically implies thoughts of artificial hormones, however. Only a few are familiar with natural methods or other fertility regulation methods.

Quit adopting external hormonal substances and trust your body's natural ways instead. Quite often, this is sufficient to conceive a child. Besides, the fact that these methods are non-hormonal can be used at any age, etc. should be pointed out here. "The rhythm method," in which the fertile phase is calculated based on basal body temperature rise, is widely known. The symptothermal method, the Billings method, and long-term protection through breastfeeding can also be cited here. Most of these methods are cited in conjunction with natural family planning. The term "natural family planning" implies that the method must be tied in with children in order to be of interest to a man. However, dosal family planning just means that a couple plans a pregnancy without taking artificial hormones to prevent pregnancy. Once the decision to have fewer or no children is made, it also stands to reason to

just plan fewer or no children using natural methods of
birth control.

4. Common Birth Control Myths

There are indeed anecdotal reports and small, short-term studies that suggest some women have experienced the symptoms of weight gain caused by birth control. Because there are different types of birth control that use different hormones and administration methods, there are varying factors to consider: 1) Many birth controls mimic natural hormones. 2) Natural hormone variations are known to affect weight. 3) Because hormones can naturally affect weight, they were likely implicated in some of the potential birth control-related weight gain reports in early studies. However, how birth control specifically is supposed to work in relation to weight is not entirely clear. No two women's bodies are alike—if hormonal shifts can naturally cause weight gain, then for anyone there can be fat held in different places throughout a woman's life.

Recent studies have shown no consistent relationship between birth control and weight gain. One report from the American College of Obstetricians and Gynecologists notes that progestin—progesterone's pharmaceutical equivalent—is one of the more widely used forms of hormonal birth control. Intrauterine devices (IUDs), contraceptive implants, and medroxyprogesterone acetate (Depo-Provera) all mostly use progestin as the active ingredient. The results from a six-year study showed that women who used a Levonorgestrel IUD for six months weighed about 2.5 pounds less on average than women who used the copper IUD over about five years. The copper

IUD is the only non-hormonal option that affects periods and acts as a birth control in the same way as hormonal IUDs and implants, whereas with ParaGard copper may induce heavier and crampier periods while Skyla can cause lighter or absent ones.

Myth 1: Birth control causes weight gain.

4.1. Myth 1: Birth Control Causes Weight Gain

The relationship between birth control and weight can be complex. For instance, a study of more than 600,000 women found weight gain was common among all women (including younger women, who are those most likely to start birth control) but did not find an association between weight gain and the use of the combined contraceptive pill. A 2015 retrospective analysis of pelvic exams from 52 patients in their 20s using the contraceptive ring found that after 6 months, 71% had gained weight.

An additional review in 2019 looking at randomized, controlled trials also found that "weight gain must be correctly informed to women requesting the use of one of these hormonal contraceptives: it could actually occur, but it seems not to be directly associated with either drugs."

A more recent review conducted with electronic databases up to February 2021 and the Cochrane Central Register of Controlled Trials (CENTRAL), two clinical trials registers, and five grey literature sources also found that adding "the results of this updated review provide evidence that does not support the belief that combined hormonal contraceptives cause weight gain, and suggest that confounding factors may be contributing to concerns about weight change amongst users."

Studies have shown that changes in weight are not directly related to the use of birth control. A 2014 review from the Cochrane Collaboration examining evidence from 49 trials concluded that while combined birth control methods may result in a small amount (less than or equal to 0.15 kg) of weight gain, the changes in weight had been shown to have no significant clinical effect. This small amount of weight gain was across various different forms of birth control, including the pill, patch, and ring.

5. Scientific Evidence on Birth Control

In matters of fertility control, what do we know to be true? A four-part series in the US has compiled and reviewed information on safer contraceptive use, the security of different contraceptive methods, and what we know about the effects of contraception. All four documents, as well as searchable spreadsheets of contraceptive data, are available online. Each report and summary reviews the sources and grading of the data upon which it is based. An associated literature database, which specifies the time period and source of each article, includes additional, or more recent than the search for the series, studies sorted by contraceptive method and subject. Available at [website removed], the web-based searchable database includes free full citations, grading criteria, a summary of the study results, and free full text of the study when available.

There is a wealth of scientific evidence guiding contraceptive practice. Studies combine published studies, expert consensus, and laboratory research, and then draw them all together. Such studies often receive valuable contributions from end-users in disagreements between clinicians, where various options seem equally appropriate. In this review, data were identified and surveyed from a variety of peer-reviewed and gray literature studies, funded by relevant government agencies and other organizations.

5.1. Research Studies and Findings

Conclusive scientific evidence is the gold standard of research for determining what works and what does not to prevent pregnancy. Scientists and medical professionals - given the ethical responsibility to protect individuals, including those not yet born - rely on conclusions from such research studies and expose their results to peer review. Ideally, these conclusions would be accepted by other concerned professionals and disseminated in ethical practices to inform and ensure the welfare and reproductive health of millions of individuals worldwide. Therein lies the idealistic goal of research promoting the highest order of legitimacy and the credentials of any argument surrounding the deployment or nondeployment of contraception.

Combatting prejudiced and biased perspectives related to contraception, the ensuing sections charted scientific evidence on a range of different scientific findings related to different methods of contraception. However, it should be accentuated here that the methods of contraception portrayed in these studies are from the time of research, and new types of contraceptive mechanisms have been developed since then. As one of the most important sources of birth control information, these types of studies do not cover other relevant findings (e.g., surgical methods, male birth control). While debunking those erroneous beliefs is important, this should not diminish the salience of evidence-based information, which has the potential to influence and educate millions of people planning to have children. Research topics include IUDs and vasectomy compared to abortion, IUD in young nulliparous women, the impact of oral contraceptives on cervical carcinogenesis, protection against HPV and warts achieved by condom use, reasons given for contraceptive choice, attitudes to postcoital contraception, condom use and reinfections in men after chlamydia treatment, as well as knowledge, attitudes and practice of Norwegian gynecologists regarding emergency contraception.

6. Importance of Access to Birth Control

This site updates regularly with new information about the content of this briefing paper included in this introduction and about specific topics such as the effects and risks of hormonal contraceptives, the history of Fertility Awareness-Based Methods, using condoms safely and effectively, and more. Access to birth control (fertility control) has a tremendous impact on people's well-being, including the ability to make choices that follow their reproductive goals. The capacity to access contraceptive technologies directly influences the likelihood of becoming parents, not becoming parents, reducing the risk of unsafe induced abortion, reducing net fertility, and spacing and timing births at women's physiological capacity. One of the most effective qualities of modern contraceptive technology is the ability to plan or delay childbearing. In other words, it affects individual and couples' pregnancy intentions and highlights the broader value of reproductive autonomy. To appreciate birth control technologies and options it is important to first understand the basic process of reproduction.

Gaining accurate information about birth control methods dispels the fear-mongering that often drives misinformation while also making it easier to gain empathy for the individual experiences of those who seek the option that is best for them. Outreach for Abortion Rights has compiled a selection of brief articles that detail the history, use, effects, risks, benefits, and non-contraceptive uses of a variety of birth control methods. Work featured at this conference has also considered how using birth control should not be treated as an isolated behavior, separate from larger life goals and values. We have explored how, to be effective, a birth control method must, on some level, align with an individual's or couple's reproductive goals, including: being childfree (not parents), having 1 or more children, giving birth or adopting, not giving birth or adopting (in the case of abortifacients), or carrying a pregnancy. This briefing paper continues this work.

6.1. Impact on Reproductive Health

Access to birth control not only shapes pregnancy intentions and outcomes but also has many other knock-on effects. One important analysis, for example, found that access to birth control was the number one predictor of whether low-income women would realize their education and career goals. These kinds of analyses seem to suggest that ensuring increased access to birth control might have a positive effect on several of the indicators of societal readiness for conception that Chapter 2 highlights. Access to birth control also has health as well as individual and societal autonomy benefits. In countries where abortion is legal, access to contraception has been an important part of creating spaces where abortion rates have decreased over time. Even in hopes of being able to strive towards a procreative future, which is a valuable part of what it means to be alive, it is important to provide options to people should they need them. Ensuring that these options are exempt from barriers to access will reduce disparities in access to healthcare and distress and risk. Preventing unintended pregnancies can save the U.S. alone billions of dollars annually in potential Medicaid costs.

Unintended pregnancy and the number of children a woman has impact a host of reproductive health indicators, including child and maternal mortality, fetal and infant health, and child nutritional status. In countries with the least access to modern contraceptives, more than 70% of the decline in fertility rates between the early 1960s to the early 2000s was due to contraception. This reduction in fertility saves the lives of many families and provides them with a range of human development advantages.

Unintended pregnancy is also an important healing, care-seeking, and medical recovery issue for women who have experienced violence, including sexual violence. Ensuring that sexually active women who choose to become pregnant have effective, affordable means to do so, without needing to forego an alternative if they have a health risk, is the cornerstone of many WHO recommendations. Pregnancy planning can also ensure that men and gender-expansive people have access to reproductive health services to help them support their partners.

7. Cultural and Societal Perspectives on Birth Control

Americans too have complicated feelings about birth control. Despite the fact that the majority of sexually active women and men have used a form of contraception, the contraceptive pill has been in the news for years, and a litany of lawsuits have been brought against its creators for health concerns. Though these cases serve as a reminder of the health risks involved with the birth control shot and the pill, they ultimately do not alter how the majority of women and young people view the importance of birth control. They see it as vital to promote self-reliance, personal liberty, open-mindedness, and sexual satisfaction. Numerous forms of contraception are also utilized for health and therapeutic reasons, such as period regulation, endometriosis, fibroids, PMDD, and acne management.

On the opposite end of the spectrum, the Humanist community has no rules or limitations. They focus on personal conscience, and in the absence of an anthropomorphic deity figure, they are able to rationalize their choices of birth control based on what they believe is best for their well-being and future.

Stemming from the power base that each religion holds in different cultures of the world, values, and morals on which they are founded, each religion holds a unique standpoint on birth control—many of which change over time, with dialogue with science, necessity, and ever-changing perspectives of society. For example, within the Judeo-Christian tradition, historically, scriptures from the Bible, popes of the Catholic Church, and other religious leaders have declared contraceptive use and all end of life birth prevention to be a sin.

For the most part, though, devout religious beliefs will have no bearing on a person's contraception use. For those who want to believe that contraceptives are just too evil, the statistics prove otherwise. According to the Family Planning New Zealand, about 100% of Catholic women in New Zealand use contraception. In the United States, Planned Parenthood says that 98% of Catholic women use contraception at some point or another. Globally, a similar number of Catholics - 98% - use contraception as well, according to World Health Organization numbers. It is important to remember that there are no records of how many people in America give up their Christianity - or upbringing thereof - to use contraception. Many women ultimately decide to have only one child, a choice that has real-world consequences as well.

The debate concerning contraception and religious views is a little more convoluted than it needs to be. Many large Christian sects promote the "Natural Family Planning" method, as well as other radical sects which promote "Quiverfull" (Natural Family Planning with a quiverful of children). "As arrows are in the hand of a mighty man, so are the children of the youth. Happy is the man that hath his quiver full of them: they shall not be ashamed, but they shall speak with the enemies in the gate." (Psalms 127:3-5) or "The Pearl Method" which includes training children to be silent and compliant with physical abuse. "This breaking process we call training, and it begins in infancy. The parents are 'the rod of authority'. Train up your child for further beatings! The rod is a once-in-a-while, not an all-the-time, training tool. Never use the rod when you are angry." Advocates include the Duggar family and the Pearls. Roman Catholics, Orthodox Christians, and a fringe minority of Protestants are dogmatically anti-contraception. The Jehovah's Witnesses are also dogmatically anti-contraception, going so far as to suggest that legal regulation of anti-venereal disease medication is equivalent to a government encouraging immoral behavior.

The consequences of religion on the contraception discussion

8. Addressing Misinformation and Disinformation

It is clear that birth control misinformation and disinformation claims are rife. With evidence-based communication strategies and comprehensive sex education, it is possible to counteract such claims. With such tools in addition to removing media portrayals that reinforce these myths or misconceptions about birth control, it is feasible to communicate key messages to debunk these popular misconceptions and move our population towards comprehensive, accurate birth control use.

In order to get to the truth, it is necessary to dispel the misinformation in favor of the facts. By educating people about birth control methods in order to combat these misconceptions, it is therefore possible to arm them with accurate information. One of the more strategic ways to correct this misinformation is via targeted health communication efforts according to the strategic communication model, including through planned, evidence-driven strategies and tools used to discuss a range of reproductive health context. Part and parcel to dispelling birth control myths is the need for comprehensive sex education to enhance knowledge and combat disinformation about contraception.

It's important to recognize that birth control myths stem from misinformation - incorrect information imparted unintentionally without harm meant to be caused. Disinformation, on the other hand, is the spreading of false information meant to mislead or manipulate the opinion or actions of others. To combat these myths, both intentional and unintentional, raised here are the frustrating misconceptions and myths about contraceptives and solutions for counteracting false claims.

Typically, we respond to these messages in comments sections with a simple (albeit occasional) "This is false. Here's how we do research on what clinicians and patients agree on when it comes to pregnancy prevention. More here: [link to our research on patient and clinician agreement about pregnancy-prevention effectiveness]." Other proactive options could be available before the messaging starts, to stop it in or before it's started in its tracks. These noses under the tent could include items like a simple repository of claims and fact-checks, both for the relevant longitudinal study itself and regarding recent relevant trials in the news like the MTF study. We envision this link from our bio/some of our socials for audiences curious about us, the authors, and our work.

The research we are rolling out today builds on a previous study from the summer that aimed to identify the impact of social media messages on perceptions of birth control. That work took place over social media and used a format that allowed subjects to engage with the content as they normally would. It found that when even a brief mention of Pandora's own longitudinal research on the impact of birth control appeared in the comments section, it significantly shaped beliefs about the birth control methods themselves. Although disinformation about birth control may not be promulgated quite as widely as it has been about vaccines - a constellation of myths poised to torpedo COVID-19 vaccination campaigns and bump up the death rate like a depopulation bomb when Phase Two arrives - it's crucial to correct and vaccinate against COVID-related birth control myths early, preemptively, and thoroughly.

9. Conclusion and Key Takeaways

Bottom line: You never know someone else's situation around starting, stopping, changing or using birth control. Misunderstandings are common, but providing accurate information and addressing myths whenever possible can help combat them. Taking an accurate description of how certain types of birth control work, including how the IUD will not usually prevent you from becoming pregnant and will not be sterile. It is also important to address the fact that most healthy adults can use hormonal birth control if necessary, even if they have menstrual cycles. In this chapter, real science can help guide you on some of these topics and help guide you to your ob-gyn if you are still looking for answers or want to remove a method. The last thing we will consider? All these methods are birth control methods that work, and the best contraceptive method for you is one that you choose and feel comfortable using! Now that we've covered the storytelling, it's time for you to make the right decisions about contraception for your health and family planning!

By discussing the myths around birth control, we hope to remove some of the stigma and misunderstandings about contraceptive methods and the people who use them. Understanding birth control, conquering your fears, and talking about insurance can empower you to maintain healthy birth control practices – or to make an informed decision about starting birth control. The decision to use birth control is entirely up to you. Just like any health decision, it's important that you can make an informed decision.

9.1. Empowering Individuals with Accurate Information

Whether your decisions are limited to family-building or involve a wide variety of relationship choices, body and dimension matters, experienced or anticipated surgeries, as well as spiritual, emotional, and mental aspects, how you want to conceive is a personal preference of bodily autonomy; rather than as 'comprehensive', especially due to socio-economic limitations since Republicans are providing sex education based on fear, banning abortion after 20 weeks, and making it impossible for you to attain hormonal prevention or self-medicate with medical alternatives, our intention is to help you make safer and fully informed reproductive decisions for both your body and general health.

Birth control is complicated. We've said it before. We'll say it again. That's why we dedicate so much time and energy to this cause: because we want people to have access to accurate information in order to make the best decision possible for their individual body and needs. We know, however, that not everyone has access to the same resources or opportunities, which is why we work to address myths we hear in our local community and to replace them with as much factual information as we can. We hope that this piece will contribute to fewer myths and more fact-based decisions. Empowerment looks different for different people; we strive to do our part to meet the needs of our community by sharing what we know.

Busting Common Myths About Birth Control

1. Introduction

Each section focuses on different methods of birth control, in order to help you better understand which method may be best suited to your needs, while also dispelling many of the rumors and myths surrounding birth control. The information provided in this guide will benefit young women and men, as well as those who have been sexually active for many years. For those who are just starting their sexual journey, we hope to provide inspiration and confidence to have meaningful discussions with trusted adults and healthcare professionals. If you or your partner are young women or non-binary people with a low socioeconomic background, mental or physical health issues, First Nations, Métis, or Inuit (FNMI), living with addictions, have a sexual or gender minority identity, or from a multi-barriered community, we encourage you to check out First Steps to help you understand pathways of support and access.

The chapters this book will explore are: The Pill, Condoms, The IUD, The Shot, The Patch, The Implant, and Natural Solutions. Each one of these topics will go over a different method of birth control along with some of the common myths and truths associated with them.

It seems as though we have entered another great era of misinformation. There exist thousands of myths, many of which surround birth control, and how it may affect a person's lifestyle and health. This great guide will aim to help reveal the truth about birth control while also providing readers with the latest information on types and methods available.

1.1. Purpose of the Work

The purpose of this work is to dispel common myths about birth control and provide important information about different contraceptive options for both women in reproductive age and adolescents. I aim to provide tools for both reproductive health providers and sexually active women to prevent seeking out fertility awareness apps or changing contraceptive choices without clear knowledge of how these options really work and their potential benefits or side effects. A better understanding of the birth control issue can provide women with higher self-confidence in making a safe contraceptive choice.

Despite the efforts being done to break the misconceptions, many people still believe that certain common myths about birth control are true. Many young women do not know how birth control works, if it's safe, or if it decreases fertility, and they feel uncomfortable discussing it with healthcare professionals. Because misapprehensions about safety and benefits may lead women to use contraceptive methods inconsistently or to avoid them entirely, it is essential for healthcare professionals to be able to answer women's questions and concerns. In order to do so, this essay will aim to provide accurate information about birth control. I propose to discuss and dispel largely all the misconceptions about oral contraception pills, intrauterine devices, condoms, contraceptives during breastfeeding, and postpartum contraceptives. It is also important to understand the negative impact of these myths on

women's health, quality of life, and parenthood, which
should not be underestimated.

2. Chapter 1: Understanding Birth Control

Methods for women include abstinence, fertility awareness method (the woman tracks her menstrual cycle and avoids having sex on her most fertile days), coitus interruptus, barrier methods (consisting of male and female condoms, diaphragm or cervical cap), spermicide, hormonal methods (consisting of estrogen and progestin combinations, progestin-only pills, hormonal shots, extended cycle pills, vaginal ring, skin patch, morning after pill, and intrauterine devices), Copper T (an intrauterine device with no hormones), and female sterilization (a surgical technique that prevents the egg from reaching the uterus).

Methods for men include condoms, outercourse (consisting of not having vaginal sex), pull-out method (consisting of moving the penis out of the woman's vagina before ejaculation), and vasectomy (a surgical procedure that prevents sperm from reaching the semen).

The etymology of birth control dates back to the early 19th century, and since then, it has defied words such as child prevention, contraception, family planning, responsible parenthood, fertility control, sexual health, and reproductive rights. Simply put, birth control, or contraception, is a method, device, or drug used to prevent pregnancy. The mechanisms of action are to stop sperm from entering the egg, to inhibit ovulation, to cause the uterine lining to thin, and to cause the uterine lining to thicken. It's important to remember that abstinence is the only certain way to prevent pregnancy. There are various types of birth control methods, different for men and women:

2.1. Definition and Types of Birth Control

A method of birth control is assigned to either: hormonal, intrauterine, permanent, non-prescription, emergency, fertility awareness, condom, sterilization, or barrier. Hormonal methods include over-the-counter birth control pills, and require a doctor's prescription. Common "pill types" include estrogen/progestin combinations, low-dose progestin products, erasing menstrual cycles, estrogen-free pills, and placebos. Over-the-counter hormonal births slow/stop ovulation, causing the endometrium to stay thin, and moving the cervical mucus. The mucus near the time of ovulation may become thick, allowing the sperm to swim through to reach the egg. Luteinizing hormone stopping may be used with other birth control methods for emergency contraception in cases of sexual assault, condom breakage, or when anchor methods have failed. Hormonal preparations have a failure rate of 1.37% with perfect use and a typical use failure rate of 7%. Collaborating methods with spermicide, the Kezierski in 2014 intrauterine insert, and the lactinex suppository demonstrate no failed prevention of impregnation in over 4,000 acts of coitus.

Birth control, also known as contraception, is the use of methods or devices to prevent pregnancy. It works by interrupting ovulation and preventing the male reproductive cells from reaching the female reproductive cells. An estimated 51% of pregnancies in the United States are unintended. Family planning is amongst the 10 great public health achievements of the 20th century. Together with condom education and distribution, hormonal birth control is one of the most used birth control methods in the United States. The types of birth control include: coitus interruptus, emergency contraception, fertility awareness, condoms, hormonal, intrauterine, permanent, barrier, and sterilization methods, along with non-prescription and prescription methods.

3. Chapter 2: Myths vs. Facts

Myth: Some pills are better than others. Fact: With so many birth control pills on the market, how can a woman be sure that the pill she is taking is right for her? Some pills, in addition to preventing pregnancy, have a health benefit. With all of this information, a woman may feel overwhelmed when deciding which pill to use. It's best to work with a trusted healthcare provider who can help you decide.

Myth: Birth control methods are dangerous and lethal to a woman's health. Fact: Today's methods of birth control are safe and effective for most women. If any of the birth control methods listed in this booklet are dangerous or harmful to your health, it will be stated in the description of the method. Any medication, not just birth control medications, may cause side effects that can interfere with a woman's life.

Myth: Women and men of childbearing age spend approximately 30 years trying not to get pregnant. Fact: The average woman spends about five years trying to get pregnant, pregnant, or postpartum. A woman who is sexually active and not trying to get pregnant but not using a contraceptive method has more than a 90 percent chance of becoming pregnant in one year.

In this chapter, each of the following myths is presented and followed immediately by the facts so that you can consider your birth control options with accurate information.

3.1. Myth: Birth Control Causes Weight Gain

Differing forms of birth control exist. Because of this, some forms of hormonal birth control lead to greater weight gain than others. Premenstrual Syndrome, contraception, PCOS, and financial uncertainties are things people discuss when they want to avoid birth control. Fruits and veggies are featured in all meals and snacks for individuals who are trying to get in form, or it can be difficult to do so if the variety of nutrients is tampered with. When mixing nutrients into your diet, you need to weigh protein, fiber, and fat to make your meals more convenient. Experts do not think that weight gain is largely linked to it. Hormonal birth control choices may have the property that works right for a person better.

As with many other difficult personal tasks, weight gain can be a cause for confusion. Whenever a female takes contraception, weight gain is often blamed on it. People who don't use birth control often put on weight. Some people have an intimate knowledge of contraception, so they would avoid it. According to a 2020 investigation, about 58% of respondents thought this was right because hormonal birth control was causing them to gain weight. A review of the scientific evidence found that they were incorrect. Meal, salt content, metabolism, and frailty were not affected by these contraceptives, according to a report written for the FDA. Hormones don't have an effect on someone's appetite, and they don't have an appetite-controlling capacity.

3.2. Myth: Birth Control is Only for Women

Progestin shots stop ovaries from releasing eggs and thin the lining of the womb. Combined birth control pills and the extended cycle (regulate when you menstruate), and patch and ring are all hormonal contraceptive options for "anybody who could get pregnant", meaning for men, this includes womb owners and prostate owners. Combined methods use both estrogen and progesterone hormone and may be more effective at preventing pregnancy than a minipill.

Long-acting reversible contraceptives (LARCs) work for ovary owners and prostate owners. Progestin implants (a matchstick-sized rod with hormones) and progestin IUD (an intrauterine device) both control when ovaries release eggs, stop sperm from reaching eggs, thicken cervical mucus to block sperm from entering the womb, and thin the womb lining, making it hard for a fertilized egg to implant. Copper IUD releases a small amount of copper into the womb, stops sperm from reaching the egg, thickens cervical mucus to block sperm from entering the womb. It may also prevent the implantation of a fertilized egg by altering the lining of the uterus.

Myth: Only women take birth control. That's just not true. Birth control includes a range of options, several of which are for people of any or all genders, so don't assume only a female partner should be the one in charge of birth control. People of any gender can take hormonal or IUD options as well as use barrier methods, fertility-based methods, or be sterilized.

3.3. Myth: Birth Control Leads to Infertility

If you are thinking about starting or stopping contraception, it is important to speak with a health professional. There are many birth control options and individual needs should be examined. Women with dysmenorrhea, heavy menstrual periods, or endometriosis, who have abnormal reproductive organs, bleed easily, or take medications that slow blood clotting, are at greater risk of developing pain or bleeding after taking the morning-after pill Levonorgestrel. Women under the age of 18 may require a prescription by a healthcare provider.

Thankfully, this is a big misconception. Birth control intervention does not affect the natural progression of ovulation. Thus, if you discontinue birth control, your rate of pregnancy should not differ. Research has found contraception does not decrease fertility. In fact, a woman's ability to conceive after stopping hormonal birth control will not differ when compared to a woman who never started birth control. However, depending on the birth control method used, your natural ovulation cycle may not return to a steady level right away. This is why doctors may encourage patients to stop taking contraception a few months before planning to become pregnant. In addition, it may take some time after stopping birth control for hormone levels to return to normal. Thus, a return to normal ovulation occurs respecting a female's health and age.

3.4. Myth: Birth Control is 100% Effective

In clinical and published research, pregnancy prevention rates focus on the use of each method within 1 year of consistent, perfect use, when available. It is also worth mentioning that birth control options, apart from abstaining, can help prevent pregnancy by providing an efficient and relatively easy and quick uptake and withdrawal in the event a baby is desired. Also, notice that a multi-section answer may be more appropriate to cover the depth and range of a topic, rather than repeating information.

Typical-use pregnancy rates out of 100 women per year include: - Implant (Nexplanon or Implanon) - 0.2 percent - Intrauterine Device (IUD) - 0.2-0.8 percent - Injections - 6 percent - Birth control pills - Typical-use 7 percent, but if taken perfectly (used at the same time each day and every day without missing any), close to 0 - Birth control patches - 7 percent - Vaginal birth control ring (NuvaRing) - 7 percent - Birth control shot - 6 percent - Withdrawal - 22 percent - Female condoms - Typical-use 21 percent, but if used perfectly close to 5 percent - Condoms - Typical-use 13 percent, but if used perfectly close to 2 percent

Birth control is used as a way for women and men to prevent unwanted pregnancy, and each body is unique. Effective use of birth control and pregnancy prevention options can depend on factors such as consistency of use, duration of use, and individual biological reactions or responses to the specific method used. Like any medical intervention, birth control options will have different effects and should be selected with the help of a physician or provider. Pregnancy rates will vary depending on the methods and individuals using them, but below are some breakdowns of typical use effectiveness.

3.5. Myth: Birth Control is Only Used for Preventing Pregnancy

Non-hormonal methods of birth control include the copper intrauterine device (IUD) and the hormonal IUD, which is also used to treat painful periods or reduce menstrual blood flow when taken as a daily pill, patch, or ring. The non-hormonal copper IUD can provide emergency contraception if inserted within 5 days of unprotected sex, but it also provides ongoing pregnancy protection for up to 12 years after it is properly inserted. Other benefits of the IUD include the provision of long-term continuous birth control over 3-10 years depending on the product, and it is the most effective method of emergency contraception when placed within 5 days of unprotected sex.

Hormonal methods are birth control options that use estrogen and/or progestin to manipulate the female's menstrual cycle, thereby stopping ovulation to prevent pregnancy. However, they can also have several non-contraceptive benefits and are used to treat painful periods, regulate a menstrual cycle, prevent premenstrual syndrome (PMS) or symptoms of premenstrual dysphoric disorder, manage symptoms of polycystic ovarian syndrome (PCOS), help clear acne, reduce menstrual flow, lower the risk of female reproductive cancers, and reduce symptoms of perimenopause, such as hot flashes. The use of these methods should be discussed with a healthcare professional to determine which method may best help to manage these medical conditions. Additionally, those who wish to use it for non-contraceptive benefits and prevent pregnancy should use it in conjunction with a second method of birth control (like the condom).

When considering birth control options, it is assumed that birth control is merely used to prevent pregnancy. While this is the most common use of birth control methods, there are also several benefits of birth control methods beyond contraception.

4. Chapter 3: Debunking Misconceptions in Different Cultural Contexts

Australia is, by comparison, relatively youth oriented and laid-back with a pragmatic culture. This has very interesting implications for the practical 'truths' and beliefs about birth control. Bulgaria, on the other hand, has gone through a minute technologisation within the past decade. This has allowed for a resurgence of traditional values of motherhood which pervade the language and attitude surrounding birth control. In the chapter, we will illustrate how the social, historical and cultural context will determine the myths used as the basis of the research and how these might be dispelled.

In the current chapter, we aim to focus on the differences and subtleties of some of the myths found in our research in Australia and Bulgaria. This will be placed against the broader social and cultural background of the lives of women within each of these countries, to give a comprehensive view of attitudes to and myths about birth control. Our work in these countries complements the work from the UK and Malaysia since it draws out different experiences and perceptions.

The previous chapters have portrayed the prevalence of myths about birth control. But how much do these myths vary in different cultural contexts? An assumption that has been made is that the myths used by family planning organisations serve the same purpose for women regardless of socio-economic or ethnic background and that women perceive and react to these in similar ways. The results from the first two chapters make plain that this is certainly not the case. Nevertheless, it is important to underscore the common elements, which suggest that for many thousands of women the myths may well have an important effect. Thus their incorporation into information giving could be key in debunking them.

Hazel Thornton, Shelley Burnham, Jill Astbury.

4.1. Cultural Myths and Realities

Romani and Irish Travelers: These people have been consistently characterized by the people around them as hyper-fertile. This concept is rooted in the historical belief that certain groups of people are "wasteful" or "promiscuous" breeders, and have more children and spouses than is good for society. In reality, fertility varies in every population. Most people, regardless of race or culture, have one or two sexual partners in their life. From a genetic point of view, the human race is no less fertile now than it was before. Irish Travelers and Romani have people of different ages within their communities like any other society, and children from those unions just like others do.

Cultural Mythologies and Realities Italy/Greece and the Mediterranean: There is a common belief in the Mediterranean that some people are able to have children and others are not, so birth control is not a big deal. This is not really the case; most people in all cultures can conceive normally. High rates of contraception use in poor areas are not due to an inability to conceive, but a very real fear of pregnancy. In societies where women are subject to constant demands for intercourse wanted by their male partners, birth control is very important to avoiding constant pregnancy and childbirth that can lead to illness or even death.

For centuries, women have been accessing birth control and other forms of fertility control to be able to make personal decisions about reproduction and family. That said, many cultural myths persist about birth control and the choices women make. It is worth noting that these are general mythologies found in many cultures over time and place, and as continuing research unfolds, we are beginning to understand how different this topic seems when approached from the perspective of people in other places and traditions.

5. Chapter 4: Addressing Common Concerns and Questions

The information provided below should help allay many of the commonly held fears associated with side effects, methods of action, safety, bleeding, infertility, and sexually transmitted infections. It's worth keeping in mind that every drug has some "side effects" and that taking any drug, even an OTC drug like a simple pain reliever, always amounts to a risk-benefit calculation. There is such a thing as a serious side effect. Moreover, contraceptive drugs are affected by all drugs, which require consideration of the issues of polypharmacy and potential drug interactions. Also, CR's work on this issue has consistently shown that many women generally think of "safety" in terms of longer-term effects; accordingly, it is precisely these evolving issues on which this chapter endeavors to focus. And when thinking about studies pertaining to safety, it's important to remember that many of the studies that have been done are too small to detect evidence of an effect.

Many people, including both current users of these methods and those who have never considered using them, have similar concerns and questions about LARCs. This chapter tries to provide detailed, evidence-based answers to some health-related and other concerns that some people have about both LARCs and hormonal contraception more generally. It attempts to provide responses that are designed to reassure women and help them make better decisions about whether LARCs are right for them. The goal is to explain the issues in sufficient detail so that women can discuss their concerns with a knowledgeable and sympathetic provider and read the scientific literature in order to learn more. However, for those principal arguments that are only mentioned briefly here, the interested reader is urged to pursue the cited reading.

This is not to say that birth control methods do not have side effects. Most of them do, especially those which contain hormones. Even though all methods on the market are FDA approved, when it comes to medications there are usually pros, cons, and potential side effects. Though these side effects are common, much of the time they dissipate with time as the body becomes more used to the medication's presence. However, decreasing such risk includes some form of an additional method of protection to reduce this risk if you would like to use such protection.

Overall, the safety outlook of using birth control is rather positive. While some types carry an array of potential side effects, including the implant and IUD, they again present some attractive features and prove to be rather safe most of the time. It should also be noted that some birth control methods use hormones while others don't, and this may prove to be beneficial and important in addressing many of the concerns that individuals may have.

A recurring concern that many individuals have about birth control entails whether the method is both safe and what the side effects might be. The side effects associated can depend on the type as well as the individual, and knowing in advance what they might entail can be a real benefit. Finally, there are segments of the public who are worried about meeting with a doctor to get birth control methods as well due to the ticker of potential risks. Many people wonder if birth control is healthy, and the short answer is yes.

6. Chapter 5: Conclusion and Key Takeaways

Getting down and dirty with the yeast, we debunked the idea that all yeast infections are the result of birth control use and estrogen levels in "libtard" cities. Lastly, and probably my most ambitious task, we tackled the idea that birth control is just there to make sex consequence free. Or rather, the concept that birth control distorts the natural reality of life by attempting to separate the "two meanings of the conjugal act" (as quoted by Pope Paul VI, in the Year of Our Lord, 1968). Besides the research and the mythbusting, what we have gathered from this essay is that debunking sexual myths that people have about the pill and the women who take it is a messy game of whack-a-mole that will quite possibly last as long as we do. Dominant views of sex, birth control, and women are built so cleanly into our society, secured, that they put themselves outside of the reach of rational argumentation. Holy mother of Christ, I just cited a Pope. Here, boys, here's a meninist merit badge.

So, as we wrap up, let's do a brief recap of the myths this essay has debunked based on research. First, we discussed the myth that the pill ruins women's hormones - this is a claim that has not been supported by science. Next, we focused on the effect of birth control on weight - this is a controversial one because there are women who experience weight gain on the pill and I don't want to dismiss their experiences. That said, the pill's hormones should not cause inherent weight gain. Third, we looked at the myth that the pill is for controlling periods. Though hormonal contraceptives often lighten periods, this is not their primary function. Fourth, we dived into the claim that condom companies add a substance to irritate the vagina.

In conclusion, let us break down the myths and the facts that dispel the false claims circling contraception. Myth 1: The hormonal IUD is unsafe for teens and women who have not had children. Reality: There are no absolute contraindications for IUD use among teens and women who have not had children. Myth 2: The copper IUD is not a good option for women with heavy menses. Reality: Studies have found the copper IUD to improve menstrual bleeding among women with heavy menses. Myth 3: The IUD is not a good option for single women. Reality: Women of all reproductive ages and relationship statuses can use IUDs safely. Myth 4: IUDs and implants can cause infertility. Reality: These methods do not cause infertility. Myth 5: Many patients are not "good candidates" for IUDs and implants. Reality: Most people can use IUDs and implants without complications. Myth 6: Inserting IUDs and implants can cause complications if an infection is present. Reality: We can insert these methods safely and promptly, even if an infection might be present. Myth 7: Women need a fertility test before choosing an IUD. Reality: Some healthcare providers inaccurately require patients to have a fertility test before getting an IUD or advise them to switch methods if they're interested in becoming pregnant within a year. This leaves many women uninformed or misinformed about contraception, dispelling commonly held beliefs and/or fears. Much unearthing needs to occur to dismantle the myths that were demystified.